Open Water Sport Diver W

Open Water Sport Diver Workbook

Richard A. Clinchy III, BS, Editor

Emergency Medical Resources
Plantation, Florida

Glen Egstrom, PhD, Associate Editor

Underwater Kinesiology Laboratory
University of California, Los Angeles
Los Angeles, California

Lou Fead, Associate Editor

Autnor, *The Easy Diver*
Miami Shores, Florida

Fifth edition

A Mosby—Jeppesen Product

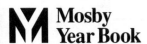
Mosby
Year Book

St. Louis Baltimore Boston Chicago London Philadelphia Sydney Toronto

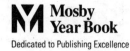

Mosby Year Book

Dedicated to Publishing Excellence

Executive Editor: Richard A. Weimer
Developmental Editor: Rina A. Steinhauer
Project Supervisor: Lilliane Anstee

Fifth edition

A Mosby—Jeppesen Product

Copyright © 1992 by Mosby–Year Book, Inc.

A Mosby imprint of Mosby–Year Book, Inc.

Printed in the United States of America

Mosby–Year Book, Inc.
11830 Westline Industrial Drive, St. Louis, Missouri 63146

92 93 94 95 96 AL/PC/PC 9 8 7 6 5 4 3 2 1

Acknowledgments

Reviewers, models, and others providing assistance for the Sport Diver project:

Divi Bahamas Beach Resort & Country Club, Nassau

Peter Hughes Diving, Nassau: Peter Hughes, Craig Burns, Harry Ward, Alan and Diana Roberts, Tony McKinney, Errol Lloyd, Andrew Higgs, Sean Lowe, and Wemzel Nichols

Orbit Marine Sports, Pompano Beach, Florida: Bob Good, Marty Knickle-Good, Patrick McKinzey, Mark Reamy

Divers Den, Ft. Lauderdale, Florida: Gary Smith, Dave Smalling, Bernardo Andrade

Samuel T. Scott, Arlington, Virginia

Paul Auerbach, MD, Vanderbilt University Medical Center, Nashville, Tennessee

William Cline, Dallas, Texas

Sharon Donovan, Moss Beach, California

Tom Griffiths, EdD, Pennsylvania State University, State College, Pennsylvania

Hammersmith International Inc., San Jose, California: Steven J. Hammersmith, Beth M. Hammersmith, Charles Chavtur, and Paul Allen Andersen

Jack Hezlep, Jeppesen Sanderson, Englewood, Colorado

Mary Jane Lewis, Dalia Jakubauskas, Stephanie Payne, Renee Roberts, Darrold Garrison, Diana DeNegre, Steve Hansen, Jeff Parker, Matt Stout, Seth Klein

Equipment manufacturers:

Ikelite Underwater Systems, Indianapolis, Indiana

Oceanic USA, San Leandro, California

Submersible Systems, Inc., Huntington Beach, California

Orca Industries, Inc., Toughkenamon, Pennsylvania

Force Fins, Santa Monica, California

Additional photography:

Dick & Nancy Clinchy, Jeff Bozanic, Matt McDermott, Ikelite Underwater Systems

Artwork:

Allan Thompson

Front cover:

Photograph by Ed Robinson/Tom Stack & Associates

PREFACE

Open Water Sport Diver Workbook is designed to supplement classroom instruction and water training under the guidance of a qualified instructor. After reading a chapter in the *Open Water Sport Diver Manual*, the student should complete the corresponding workbook exercise. With few exceptions, the answers use the completion format of recall. This type of question has been found to provide greatest retention when used as a testing methodology. The student should simply circle or write in the correct answer directly on the workbook sheet in the space provided. For example:

1. The body uses oxygen and produces
   a. Nitrogen
   b. Carbon dioxide
   c. Carbon monoxide
   d. Nitrous oxide
2. When wearing fins, walk BACKWARD.

Each self-study exercise tests and reinforces the student's comprehension of the material covered in the manual. The exercises also focus attention on practical application of the information contained in the manual, on problem-solving techniques and methods in real life diving situations.

Whether the workbook is used as a study guide, quiz book, or for instructor evaluation of student comprehension, the exercises should be completed soon after reading the manual both to test and to effectively reinforce the material covered in the manual.

After completing an exercise, students should either grade it themselves using the answers given at the back of the workbook, or they should remove the perforated sheet from the workbook and give it to the instructor for grading (whichever is preferred by the instructor). Each student should ensure that his or her name, date, and class number are clearly written on the appropriate pages of the workbook. Each completed exercise can be retained by the instructor for a permanent record of the student's achievement.

The safe diving practices in the back of the workbook should be read, understood, and signed. The signed standards should be given to the instructor at the completion of the course.

An evaluation form also is included at the back of the workbook to give the student an opportunity to comment confidentially on the course. The student is encouraged to fill out the form and return it to the instructor at the completion of the course.

Contents

Chapter 1

_____ _____ _____

NAME   DATE   CLASS NO.

1. Three items make up the basic equipment of the skin diver. They are:
   a. _Mask_
   b. _Fins_
   c. _Snorkel_

2. Low-volume masks are designed to keep the air space within the mask _Small_.

3. Large-volume masks are probably best suited for _Scuba_ divers since they have more air available for clearing the mask.

4. Two features of silicone compound as a mask material are:
   a. Silicone is _hypoallergenic_.
   b. It is resistant to _Etia aft ozone_ deterioration.

5. Two specific things mentioned in the book that may cause rubber to deteriorate are:
   a. Exposure to _heat_
   b. _Skin_   _oil_

6. The two most significant considerations in purchasing a mask are _fit_ and _comfort_.

7. The glass used in a mask should be _____.

8. Two features considered to be important regarding the band surrounding the lens are:
   a. Made of _____ materials.
   b. Be _____ to allow for re-placement.

9. Mask strap buckles should be _____ and have _____ _____ de-vices.

10. The purge valve, if included in your mask, will assist you in _____ _____ from the mask.

11. The feature of a mask that helps to provide a good seal is the _____, which has a double seal.

12. When putting a mask on or repositioning it under water be sure to _____ _____ in order to avoid the irritation of water being forced into your nostrils as the mask is positioned.

13. Without defogging solution or some form of wetting solution, warm humid air will _____ on the inner surface of your mask lens.

14. One method to prevent ear squeeze is to be sure you can equalize _____ you dive.

15. If, for some reason, you cannot equalize your ears you should _____ your dive.

16. There are two types of fins. They are:
    a. _____-_____ fins
    b. _____-_____ fins

17. Select the type of fins that usually come in small, medium, large, and extra-large sizes:
    a. Full-foot fins
    b. Open-heel fins

18. Three factors to consider when choosing fins are:
    a. Diver _____
    b. _____ strength
    c. Diving _____

19. If diving from a boat in warm water, select the best fin choice:
    a. Full-foot fins
    b. Open-heel fins

1

20. Fins that are too loose may:
    a. _____
    b. _____
    c. Fall _____
    d. Cause _____
21. Booties worn in warm water _____ the feet when walking on rough surfaces to a dive site.
22. List the four major kicks described in the text:
    a. _____ kick
    b. _____ kick
    c. _____ kick
    d. _____ kick
23. The scuba diver can use the snorkel to _____ _____while swimming on the surface or while _____ the dive _____.
24. Snorkels are divided into two general classes: _____ and _____.
25. In selecting a snorkel, two major factors to consider are:
    a. _____ _____
    b. _____

26. Most modern snorkels allow you to adjust the position of the _____.
27. The mouthpiece material that is most comfortable and hypoallergenic is _____.
28. Methods used by divers for snorkel clearing are _____ and the _____ _____.
29. A good entry is _____, _____, and not _____.
30. The most popular feet-first entry is the _____ _____ .
31. The _____-_____ is most often used when diving from a small boat or rubber raft.
32. Making beach entries through a surf includes _____ the fins and _____ backward.
33. The feet-first surface dive is used primarily in _____.
34. After a dive, as you ascend,_____ ____ and _____ so you can see boats or other objects that may be in your path.

Chapter 2

_____   _____   _____
NAME   DATE   CLASS NO.

1. Protective suit choices are:
   a. Thin _____ _____ _____
   b. Foam-neoprene _____ _____
   c. Variable-volume _____ _____
2. Dive skins provide some _____ protection and protection from _____ and _____.
3. Water absorbs body heat _____ times faster than air.
4. Wet-suit material thicker than 1/4 inch provides increased insulation but also increases _____.
5. To provide for maintenance of warmth and comfortable movement, the most important consideration in selecting a wet suit is _____ _____.
6. Arrange the following wet suit components in the order recommended for donning (write numbers in spaces provided which indicate the order):
   _____ Fins
   _____ Mask
   _____ Weight belt
   _____ BC
   _____ Pants
   _____ Gloves
   _____ Jacket
   _____ Hood
   _____ Boots
7. No more than _____ inches of webbing should extend beyond the buckle once appropriate weights are placed on the belt.
8. To provide consistency, the buckle should be placed in such a way as to allow for _____ with the _____ hand.

9. The mask skirt, when being used with a wet-suit hood, should be seated firmly against the face _____ the hood.
10. Three features of the dry suit which keep it dry include:
    a. Seals at the _____ and _____
    b. Waterproof _____
    c. Attached _____
11. Dry suits are recommended for:
    a. Diving in _____ _____ water
    b. Extended _____ _____ in _____ cold water
12. When adjusting weights on a weight belt, add and subtract weights until you _____ _____ when you exhale completely and _____ _____ when you inhale completely.
13. The weight belt should be made of _____ _____.
14. The weight belt buckle should be easy to _____ with either hand, even when wearing gloves.
15. Vinyl coating on weights help protect _____ and _____ decks.
16. In ditching the weight belt in an emergency, you must pull it away from your waist as far as you can so you can _____ ____ _____ freely and clearly.
17. The "horse collar" BC is primarily used for _____ _____.
18. Low-profile BCs place most of the buoyancy around the _____ and under the _____, which leaves the lifting air under the water at the surface.

3

19. _____ _____ BCs are normally easier to repair if damaged.
20. _____ _____ BCs offer reduced bulk and lower drag.
21. It is recommended that you always dive with a _____

_____ _____.
22. Testing the BC for leaks is accomplished by _____ it and _____ it in the bathtub, sink, or swimming pool.

Chapter 3

1. Smaller scuba tanks are lighter and easier for _____ or _____ divers.
2. The two metals used in the manufacture of scuba tanks are _____ and _____.
3. The outside surface of all steel tanks should be _____.
4. Without correct tank markings, a tank is _____.
5. Most common scuba tanks used today are not pressurized beyond _____ psig.
6. The simple "on-and-off" valve on a scuba tank is called the _____ valve.
7. A valve equipped with a lever, sometimes referred to as a constant reserve tank valve, is called a _____ valve and is seen less frequently today in sport diving.
8. What is the item that forms the seal between the tank valve and the regulator yoke? _____
9. A backpack should be equipped with a _____-_____ fastening at the waist for easy jettisoning of the tank during rescue.
10. Check the tightness of the _____ _____ before each dive.
11. Keeping _____ out of the scuba tank is probably the single most important element of tank care.
12. When storing a steel tank retain _____ (low/high) pressure in the tank.
13. A thorough visual inspection of a tank should take place at least _____.
14. Damp air coming out of a scuba tank is _____.
15. Pure, clear air _____ _____ smell.

16. If a scuba tank is clean and dry, what should you hear with your ear next to the tank, when you turn the tank upside down? _____
17. Tanks should be hydrostatically tested every _____ years.
18. Modern regulators reduce the tank pressure to breathable pressures in _____ stages.
19. A _____ hose, _____-_____ regulator is almost the only type used in sport diving today.
20. Three factors to consider in regulator selection include _____ _____, _____, and _____.
21. The extra second stage attached to an extra low-pressure port on the first stage is called an "_____" regulator.
22. The octopus regulator provides an independent mouthpiece for emergency _____ _____.
23. The octopus also provides a backup system in case the _____ _____ _____ fails.
24. Some divers carry an entirely separate _____ and _____ stage along with its own _____ _____.
25. Utilizing a submersible pressure gauge, a diver should check tank pressure _____.
26. When rinsing the second stage, it is important not to press the _____ _____, or water may enter the air hose and contaminate it.

27. If the regulator is ever out of your mouth while underwater, _____ gently at all times!

28. Two methods to clear the second-stage regulator of water include _____ the regulator clear or pressing the _____ _____ to use tank air to clear the regulator.

29. In buddy breathing, two divers share _____ second-stage regulator for breathing.

30. During buddy breathing, the donor should maintain _____ contact with the buddy.

31. When buddy breathing, make sure both you and your buddy _____ _____ when not inhaling.

32. During the buddy breathing ascent, if either of you is not exhaling when the regulator is not in your mouth, _____ _____ _____ until exhalation is resumed.

33. Know your buddy's gear well enough to _____ and _____ it at a moment's notice.

34. Buddy pairs should agree on how they will _____ _____, what _____ to use, and what to do in case of an _____.

35. When diving, your buddy should be _____ _____ _____.

Chapter 4

_____ _____ _____

NAME   **DATE**   **CLASS NO.**

1. The _____ is the only way to assess accurately how much air you have to continue the dive.
2. The SPG should have a swivel _____, large _____, and scratch-resistant _____.
3. Develop the habit of _____ _____ your gauge, to track air _____ and _____ air supply.
4. Not all _____-_____ or _____ watches can withstand increased water pressure without damage.
5. Some diving computers and dive watches automatically activate the dive-timing mechanism as soon as your depth exceeds a preset, _____ _____ depth.
6. The four types of depth gauge include:
   a. _____
   b. _____ _____
   c. _____
   d. _____
7. The _____ gauge is the simplest and least expensive.
8. The _____ _____ _____ eliminates guesswork in determining your maximum depth after a dive.
9. All diving computers constantly monitor the diver's _____ and _____.
10. Before using a computer, read the _____ _____ thoroughly.
11. Each diver should carry his or her own _____ _____.

12. Even with a computer, _____ _____ with respect to the no-decompression limits.
13. Make only _____-_____ _____.
14. Do not exceed the computer-specified _____ _____.
15. Make a safety stop between _____ and _____ feet for _____ to _____ minutes during your ascent.
16. Always make your _____ dive first.
17. As a general rule, do not turn _____ _____ _____.
18. Know what to do in the event of computer _____.
19. Abide by the _____ after diving procedures.
20. A compass increases _____ and _____ of a dive.
21. The _____ is the easiest way to maintain a valid sense of direction.
22. A _____ compass is the least expensive and can give you a general sense of direction when diving.
23. Knowing that a compass always gives direction in terms of a 360 degree circle, indicate the following equivalents:
   a. North is _____ degrees
   b. East is _____ degrees
   c. South is _____ degrees
   d. West is _____ degrees
24. Regardless of the type of compass utilized, hold it _____ when reading.
25. A reciprocal compass course is _____ from the original course and is the course to follow to return to your point of origin.
26. _____ and _____ lean with the current.
27. _____ _____ on a sandy bottom generally run parallel to the prevailing surface waves.

7

Chapter 5

_____ _____ _____

NAME   DATE   CLASS NO.

1. A dive flag will make a diver more _____.

2. The _____ flag is white and blue with a "V" cut into the outside edge.

3. The _____ is easier to hear over wind and waves and is less tiring than shouting or waving the arms.

4. _____ _____ _____ may be activated at the beginning of a dive so that buddies can keep track of each other.

5. The diver knife or tool may be used as a:
   a. _____
   b. _____
   c. _____
   d. _____
   e. _____ - _____
   f. _____
   g. _____
   h. _____ _____

6. The primary purpose of the diver knife is to cut _____ _____ if entangled.

7. The simplest underwater light is similar to a standard flashlight except that it is _____ so as to be watertight.

8. Other lights are brighter since they utilize a _____ _____ light source.

9. Any diving light must be _____ and _____ _____.

10. Knowing water temperature helps in _____ _____ _____.

11. The data in the dive log are definitely needed for the planning of a _____ _____.

12. In addition to a certification card, the trend in the diving industry is to require a _____ as evidence of recent diving experience.

13. A waterproof, dry container should be taken on all dives with _____ and _____ _____.

14. The gear bag you select should be large enough to hold all your gear, except the _____ and _____ _____.

Chapter 6

| NAME | DATE | CLASS NO. |

1. If someone floats easily without donning equipment, the person has _____ _____.

2. If the same person tends to sink, he or she is _____ _____.

3. If the person neither floats nor sinks, he or she is _____ _____.

4. Since density of water affects buoyancy, it is easier to float in _____ _____.

5. While looking forward, objects appear 25% _____ and 25% _____ than they really are.

6. The _____ and _____ (colors) begin to be absorbed in the first 30 feet of depth.

7. Sound moves _____ times faster under water than in air.

8. _____ should be reviewed with your buddy before diving.

9. Body heat is lost at a rate _____ times faster in water than in air of the same temperature.

10. If you ever start shivering violently during a dive, _____ the dive.

Chapter 7

_____   _____ _____
                    NAME   DATE   CLASS NO.

1. Air you inhale contains about _____%
   nitrogen.
2. Nitrogen is an _____
   (chemically inactive) gas.
3. Feeling "out of breath" is a response to too
   much _____ _____
   in the blood.
4. While diving, if you feel "hungry" for air,
   immediately _____, _____,and
   _____ _____ until you
   have lost the feeling of air hunger.
5. While skin diving, never hyperventilate
   more than _____ or _____ times before a
   surface dive.
6. Three recognizable signs of panic are:
   a. A _____ -_____ look
   b. Very _____ breathing
   c. Undirected _____
7. During a dive, if you feel anxious or are
   having difficulty in any way, _____
   and _____. Relax and _____
   _____ and _____ until you
   have solved the problem and regained
   complete control.

8. Artificial ventilation is done by _____
   -to-_____ resuscitation.
9. Artificial circulation is done by external
   _____ _____.
10. The process of combining artificial venti-
    lation and artificial circulation is known as
    _____.
11. The second step in CPR is to _____
    _____ victim's _____.
12. Before initiating artificial circulation, you
    must check the victim's _____.
13. Infection risk can be minimized during
    artificial ventilation by using a _____
    _____ device.
14. Sport divers should never breathe any
    gas underwater but _____, _____,
    _____ air.
15. Fill your scuba tanks at reputable
    _____ _____ stations.

Chapter 8

_____   _____   _____
NAME   DATE   CLASS NO.

1. At sea level, ordinary air pressure is _____ psi.

2. In sea water, one atmosphere pressure is added for every _____ feet of depth.

3. In fresh water, one atmosphere pressure is added for every _____ feet of depth.

4. _____ pressure is the combination of ambient air pressure plus the pressure exerted by water.

5. In sea water at 66 feet the absolute pressure is _____ ATA.

6. According to Boyle's law, the volume of a flexible container at 2 ATA will be _____ as great as at sea level.

7. Conversely, if a flexible container is filled with air at 33 feet depth in sea water, the volume will be _____ times as great at sea level.

8. The effects of Boyle's law on the air-filled spaces in the diver's body include:
   a. _____
   b. _____
   c. _____ and _____
   d. _____
   e. _____

9. Equalization of the ears involves air passing through the eustachian tubes into the _____ _____.

10. A problem involving the air spaces in the skull connected to the nasal passages, which can result in pain if equalization does not occur, is called _____ _____.

11. If you hold your breath on an ascent, air in your lungs will expand, consistent with Boyle's law, and may result in an _____ _____, which can be life threatening.

12. The first-aid steps for treating air embolism include:
    a. Lay the victim _____ on a firm surface.
    b. Perform _____ as needed.
    c. Administer _____ _____ to the breathing diver.
    d. If CPR is being performed, _____ _____ should also be administered.
    e. Treat the victim for _____.
    f. Have the victim immediately transported to a medical facility with a _____ _____.

13. The emergency phone number for DAN is _____-_____-_____.

14. The simplest rule for preventing air embolism while diving is NEVER _____ _____ _____ while scuba diving.

15. There is a 100% increase in pressure in the first _____ feet of water. Conversely, an object's volume increases _____% between 33 feet depth in sea water and the surface, so the risk of air embolism from holding one's breath is greatest in shallow water.

16. The first step in preparing to surface is to confirm with _____ _____ that it is time to surface.

17. When you are ascending, your inflator hose should be above your _____.

18. The ascent rate recommended utilizing the U.S. Navy Diving Table is not in excess of _____ feet per minute.

19. On dives to a depth of greater than 40 feet, it is recommended that a safety stop be made for _____ minutes at a depth of between 10 and 30 feet.

20. Once you reach the surface following a dive, give the _____ sign to the boat or beach.

21. The best protection against making emergency ascents is NOT RUNNING _____ _____ _____ .

22. The least preferable form of shared air ascent is _____ _____.

23. Buoyancy in the emergency buoyant ascent is largely created by ditching your _____ _____.

Chapter 9

_____ _____ _____
NAME   **DATE**   **CLASS NO.**

1. It is suggested that sport divers limit the depth of their diving to _____ feet or less.
2. Most sport divers dive in water depths of _____ feet or less.
3. Nitrogen _____ has been known to affect divers at depths as shallow as _____ feet.
4. According to Martini's law, diving at a depth of 100 feet is roughly equivalent to drinking _____ martinis.
5. _____ toxicity will never be a problem for the sport diver who breathes clean, dry, filtered air and stays within the 100-foot depth limit.
6. Theoretically, taking partial pressures into consideration, a diver might suffer _____ _____ at a depth of 250 feet while breathing air.
7. Decompression sickness—DCS or the bends—is a result of _____ gas coming out of solution too rapidly when ambient pressure is reduced.
8. Like opening a soda bottle slowly, the secret to avoiding decompression sickness is to decompress _____.
9. Symptoms of decompression sickness are usually delayed more than _____ minutes after the affected diver surfaces.
10. Symptoms of decompression sickness will usually occur during the _____ _____ after a dive.
11. Cases of decompression sickness have been reported as late as _____ hours after the last exposure to pressure.
12. List seven signs and symptoms of decompression sickness:
    a. _____ pain

b. Skin _____
c. _____ and _____ in the extremities
d. _____ change
e. _____
f. Impairment of _____
g. _____

13. The maximum allowable bottom time for a 60-foot dive using the U.S. Navy Tables is _____ minutes.
14. List four factors that might reduce the effectiveness of the No-Decompression Limits on dive tables:
    a. _____
    b. _____
    c. _____
    d. _____
15. One condition in women which should keep them away from diving is _____.
16. The ascent rate recommended by the U.S. Navy Diving Table is _____ feet per minute.
17. The slowest ascent rate utilized by any diving computers currently on the market is _____ feet per minute.
18. Bottom time is generally described as the time from the beginning of your _____ until you begin your _____ _____ to the surface.
19. The maximum altitude at which the U.S. Navy Diving Tables may be utilized is _____ feet.
20. The minimum time you should remain out of the water before flying is _____ hours, and some authorities are advising a delay of not less than _____ hours before flying, to avoid decompression sickness.

Chapter 10

NAME   DATE   CLASS NO.

1. If a diver stays at a given depth for _____ hours, the body is said to be _____.

2. Decompression tables are designed to allow for _____ to come out of solution in the body slowly.

3. As an additional measure of safety, it is prudent if you stop for at least 3 minutes at a depth of between _____ and _____ feet on every no-decompression dive.

4. Nitrogen that may remain in solution in your body following a dive is called _____ nitrogen and must be taken into consideration during any subsequent dives.

5. Using dive tables, _____ refers to the deepest point reached at any time during the dive.

6. By U.S. Navy and most table standards, a _____ _____ is a dive that starts within 12 hours of the most recently concluded dive.

7. The diagram that might be drawn to describe a dive is called a dive _____.

8. The time elapsed between the end of one dive and the descent at the beginning of another dive is known as _____ _____ _____ and may be abbreviated as _____.

NOTE: All of the following dive table problem solutions utilize the following tables: U.S. Navy; Jeppesen version of U.S. Navy; DCIEM; NAUI; PADI. The answer key provides solutions for each of these tables. If you are utilizing a table other than those mentioned, your instructor will provide you with appropriate solutions.

9. A diver has not been diving for several days and wishes to make a first dive to a depth of 60 feet. The maximum bottom time for a 60-foot maximum depth dive is_____ minutes.

10. If the diver makes a 50-minute dive to a maximum of 60 feet, the letter group at the end of the dive is _____.

11. The diver wishes to make a second dive to a depth of 50 feet and remain at that depth for 50 minutes. The minimum surface interval before starting the second dive is _____ minutes.

12. If the diver stays out of the water for 3 hours (180 minutes) between the first and second dive, the letter group at the start of the second dive will be _____.

13. Residual nitrogen time of _____ minutes must be added to actual bottom time at the beginning of the second dive, to calculate total bottom time.

14. If the diver completes the second dive to 50 feet for 50 minutes following the 3-hour surface, the diver's letter group at the end of the second dive is _____.

15. For the table used in problems 13 through 18, the maximum altitude at which the table may be used is _____ feet.

16. For the table utilized in problems 13 through 18, the recommended maximum ascent rate is _____ feet per minute.

17. Though there is no guarantee, the primary reason for using tables is to limit your risk of getting _____ _____.

18. For the dive profile below, fill in the miss-
ing information:

Group = * Group = __ Group = __ Group = __

SIT = 2:35

Maximum
depth = 70 ft

Maximum
depth = 40

ABT = 40 min
RNT = 0 min

TBT = 40 min

ABT = 60 min
RNT = __ min

TBT = __ min

Chapter 11

_____   _____   _____

NAME   **DATE**   **CLASS NO.**

1. The oceans cover _____ % of the earth's surface.
2. Along most of the continents' coasts, the bottom gradually slopes to a depth of 600 feet, then falls away rapidly. This characteristic of the continents is called the

   _____ _____.
3. _____ is the branch of science that studies the interrelationships of living organisms and their environment.
4. _____ _____ gives a dive site its distinctive life.
5. Corals cannot withstand water temperatures much below _____ °F.
6. Layers of water in which the temperature changes significantly are called _____.
7. When the layer of surface water cools and sinks to a level where similar water temperatures exist, this shift in water is called an _____.
8. Wind blowing offshore, causing bottom water to flow in and replace the water moving away from shore, is called _____.

9. Most weather is the result of _____ interaction.
10. When airmasses with different characteristics meet, they form a _____ zone or _____.
11. The agency that observes and tracks airmasses is the _____ _____ Service.
12. Broadcasts from the National Oceanic and Atmospheric Administration, also known as _____, are heard on special weather radios and the following VHF-FM marine weather channel frequencies:
    a. _____
    b. _____
    c. _____
13. Three conditions that might indicate deteriorating weather conditions include rapid _____ build-ups, sudden _____ shifts, and _____ changes.
14. Dewpoint is the temperature to which air must be cooled to become _____ with water vapor.
15. A _____ barometer usually indicates deteriorating weather conditions.

Chapter 12

NAME   DATE   CLASS NO.

1. Tides can be thought of as _____ in the water created by the gravitational pull of the _____ and the _____.
2. When the tidal bulge approaches a coastline, the water level rises, and this creates a _____ _____.
3. When the tide changes direction, there is a period in which no vertical motion occurs. This is referred to as the _____.
4. The tidal _____ is the vertical distance between the levels of the high and low tides.
5. The sloping shore that is exposed during low tide is called the _____ _____.
6. _____ _____ is the horizontal flow of water caused by the tides.
7. Tidal current moving toward the land is called _____ current.
8. The _____ current is tidal current moving away from the land.
9. When the tidal current changes direction, there is a period when there is no horizontal movement, which is called _____ time.
10. The unceasing movements of water within the oceans are referred to as the six major _____ currents in the ocean.
11. Currents in the northern hemisphere circulate in a _____ direction. Currents in the southern hemisphere circulate in a _____ direction.
12. Waves may be generated by _____ or as a result of some _____ disturbance beneath the waters' surface.
13. How hard the wind blows is called _____.
14. _____ is known as the distance over which the wind continues to blow.
15. When the wind remains constant, the steady state reached by the water is referred to as _____.
16. Measuring from trough to crest is the _____ of a wave.
17. Measuring from _____ to _____ is the length of a wave.
18. Waves breaking away from the shore generally indicate the presence of a submerged _____ or _____.
19. The seaward movement of water which is mistakenly referred to as "undertow" is properly called _____.
20. _____ is the back-and-forth movement created when the circular energy movement within a wave reaches shallower water and is influenced by the bottom.
21. _____ currents flow parallel to the shore.
22. _____ currents flow out from the beach side of a surf zone.
23. When diving from a boat with a current present, always swim _____ the current at the beginning of the dive.
24. Especially when swimming in a current, a _____ may enable you to signal to your boat if you are swept down current.

23

Chapter 13

1. Corals are found in both _____ and _____ varieties and are related to hydroids, hydras, jellyfishes, and sea anemones.
2. Corals reproduce _____ by interacting with other corals and _____ by dividing themselves.
3. Coral is limited to _____ _____depths in _____ water.
4. Zooxanthellae are algae which have a _____ relationship with coral.
5. A large contributor to reef building is the sponge (Porifera), a form of _____.
6. The midreef is found in _____ to _____ feet of water.
7. Coral requires water temperatures above _____ °F and occurs in ocean waters between _____ °north and _____ °south of the Equator.
8. Coral reefs are found only on the _____ shores of the continents.
9. In cold ocean waters, bottom formations are made up principally of _____ and in some areas there are beds of _____.
10. Kelp is a large form of _____.
11. In the process of eating living coral, the _____ produces enough sand to cover approximately one acre yearly.
12. The main food for _____ are _____ and barnacles.
13. To diminish the risk of shark attack, do not carry _____ or _____ _____ when underwater in the ocean.
14. The habit of the _____ is to usually approach a diver to within about 4 feet and simply hang around.
15. A _____ _____ might bite you if you stick your hand into a hole in which one resides.
16. Stingray injuries can be avoided by divers if they _____ their feet when wading in shallow water having a sandy bottom.
17. Fire coral is not a true coral, and the diver should _____ all contact with it.
18. Marine life defenses include:
    a. _____
    b. _____
    c. _____
    d. _____
    e. _____
    f. _____

Chapter 14

NAME	DATE	CLASS NO.

1. Other than lakes and rivers, fresh water diving sites might include _____, _____, _____, _____ and _____.

2. Cave, cavern, wreck, and ice diving are all considered _____ environments and require specialized training far beyond basic sport diver training.

3. The Great Lakes, in the United States, contain _____ % of the world's fresh water.

4. _____ lakes are normally clear and offer the greatest freshwater diving potential.

5. _____ offer interesting freshwater diving opportunities because of their importance in early exploration, transportation, and commerce.

6. With extremely clear water and relatively warm, year-round constant water temperatures of about 72 °F, _____ and _____ offer excellent opportunities for underwater photography.

7. The _____ sunfish is a distant cousin to the ocean damselfish.

8. Four types of amphibians are _____, _____, _____, and _____.

9. Four types of reptiles are seen in North America, and three of these may be seen while diving, including _____, _____, and _____.

10. The most common and dangerous mammal encountered while diving is _____.

11. The sea cow or _____ may be found in freshwater springs and rivers in Florida, and is seriously endangered.

Chapter 15

NAME   DATE   CLASS NO.

1. When organisms live together and one might normally be prey for the other, but instead the relationship is mutually beneficial, the relationship is known as _____.

2. Dumping of _____ and _____ may not only kill marine organisms but also produces diseases and mutations.

3. _____ _____ is just one problem that may be the result of pollution and causes filter feeders, such as oysters, to become toxic.

4. The _____ often created by dredge-and-fill construction ultimately settles, killing both coral and the young of many species.

5. Ballast pumping is a major source of worldwide _____ pollution.

6. In commercial fishing, _____-_____ is a major source of the decline of some fish populations.

7. Spearfishing activities should be limited to the taking of fish for _____.

8. _____ is a process in which too many nutrients enter a body of fresh water, causing an explosive increase in plant growth.

9. "Smokestack" industry is felt to be the source of _____ _____, which most significantly affects freshwater life forms.

10. _____ is everyone's problem!

Chapter 16

1. The seas are beginning to show the effects of regional _____.
2. Killing fish simply for _____ may deplete breeding stock and unbalance the ecosystem.
3. The _____ _____ in operation is quite similar to the slingshot.
4. Two considerations in spear gun selection:
   a. Type of _____ being sought
   b. _____ in which one plans to pursue game
5. Always _____ and _____ a speargun in the water, away from others.
6. In Southern California, the sport daily limit for abalone is _____.
7. If an undersized abalone is taken and not properly returned to its habitat, it may either _____ or be _____ by predators.
8. Found crawling along the bottom, primarily in warm ocean waters, the _____ is an excellent source of food.
9. The _____ lobster is found along the U.S. west coast, throughout the Caribbean, and up the U.S. east coast as far north as Virginia.
10. The _____ lobster has larger front claws and is found in the cold waters of the northeastern United States and Canada.
11. _____ of one form or another are found virtually all over the world.
12. Successful sea-farming ventures include _____ and _____ and the cultivation of _____ and _____ beds.
13. _____ is being used as a human food supplement and as a source of minerals and vitamins.

31

Chapter 17

1. Every dive you will ever make requires some degree of _____ and preparation.

2. As a sport diver, _____ should be a regular part of your daily activities.

3. _____ is an important factor in preparing for a dive.

4. Foods that are high in _____ and _____ reduce the ability of the blood to transfer oxygen to your muscles and brain.

5. Complex carbohydrates, such as _____ _____, _____, _____, and _____ promote controlled energy absorption.

6. _____ prior to a dive is another important health and safety consideration.

7. Clear _____ before a dive is a good indication that you are adequately hydrated.

8. The following beverages increase urine output so are poor choices for hydration:
   a. _____
   b. _____
   c. _____
   d. _____

9. A woman using birth control pills should probably dive _____ relative to the dive table being used.

10. A dive _____ insures that you and your buddy have agreed and are coordinated to do the same thing underwater.

11. Once a dive objective has been selected, then the next step is to pick an appropriate dive _____.

12. List below some of the information you should secure when scouting a dive site:
    a. _____
    b. _____
    c. _____
    d. _____
    e. _____
    f. _____
    g. _____
    h. _____

13. An important part of scouting the dive site is researching the _____ services available and preparing an _____ plan.

14. Use an _____ to ensure that nothing is overlooked or forgotten.

15. Evaluation of _____ conditions is always left to the day of the dive and points to the need to always plan for an alternative dive site.

16. In planning for a dive, divers should begin monitoring weather conditions about 1 _____ before the dive.

17. Always be certain that someone not involved in your dive knows your _____ _____.

18. Plan your dive and _____ _____ _____.

19. As a safe diver, I should _____ a dive when my physical condition or that of my buddy is questionable.

20. Ascend no faster than _____ feet per minute but, more appropriately, try to keep the ascent rate to no more than _____ feet per minute.

21. Never dive below _____ feet.

Chapter 18

NAME	**DATE**	**CLASS NO.**

1. In the United States, the greatest concentration of underwater caves is in the _____.

2. Manmade caves include abandoned _____ and _____.

3. When an underground river flows near the surface and its roof caves in, a _____ is formed.

4. In a _____, the diver must be able to see natural light from the entrance at all times.

5. In cavern diving, divers must remain within _____ linear feet of the surface.

6. In cavern diving, no _____ may be passed through.

7. Water visibility in a cavern must be at least _____ feet.

8. In cavern diving, maximum depth may not exceed _____ feet.

9. No _____ diving is permitted in cavern diving.

10. Ice diving requires equipment and training similar to that of _____ diving.

11. Special training is required for wreck diving since it is very much like _____ _____.

12. Treasure may come in the form of precious metals or gems or may come in the form of _____.

13. Wreck diving for treasure involves a great deal of expense and research, while _____ can be done on a small budget.

14. Blue-water diving is conducted where the _____ is _____ than safe diving limits.

15. Blue-water diving requires good _____ _____ skills.

16. In blue-water diving a _____ _____ provides a visual reference for the divers.

17. All divers in blue-water diving are attached to the down line with a _____.

18. If you are interested in Search and Rescue diving, contact your local _____ _____ agency which can put you in touch with local units.

19. _____ is the national organization that is a source of information regarding search and rescue.

Chapter 19

NAME   DATE   CLASS NO.

1. If you are ultimately interested in sharing your excitement about diving, earning a living as a scuba _____ is a possibility you might wish to consider at a later date.

2. Because of the demand for information as diving grows, _____ and photography are fields which offer greater and greater opportunities in diving.

3. Three major areas of journalism in diving are _____, _____, and _____.

4. The best way to present the underwater world to the nondiver is through _____.

5. Light commercial work is normally defined as underwater work accomplished in a _____ amount of time or in shallow enough water so that _____ is unnecessary.

6. Finding jobs that can be completed with scuba simply requires _____.

7. To do light commercial diving, you should seek out appropriate additional _____.

8. Heavy commercial diving is the highest _____ and most _____ of all commercial diving.

9. Some aspects of heavy commercial diving include underwater _____, the use of _____ hat and _____ _____ units, as well as heavy construction techniques.

10. In order for scientific diving activities to be exempt from OSHA regulations, they must be conducted in accordance with the standards of _____ (the American Academy of Underwater Sciences).

11. Two major areas of scientific diving include _____ and _____.

Appendix A

SPORT DIVER STANDARDS FOR SAFE DIVING

AS A SAFE DIVER, I SHOULD:

Dive within my mental and physical limits

Be aware of the need for good physical conditioning in connection with scuba diving

Be aware of the effects of drugs, alcohol, tobacco, and fatty foods on my personal diving safety

Cancel dives when my physical condition or that of my buddy is questionable

Dive within the limits of my training and experience

Always dive with a certified and equally qualified buddy

Have an emergency plan prepared and at the dive site

Avoid excessive hyperventilation when breath-hold diving

Descend slowly and equalize my ears prior to and frequently during descent

Ascend no faster than 60 feet per minute but more appropriately no more than 40 feet per minute

Conduct a safety stop with my buddy at 20 feet to 30 feet for 3 to 5 minutes after every dive

Be familiar with the dive tables and how to use them

Be conservative with the dive tables

Plan the dive and follow the dive plan

AS A SAFE DIVER, I SHOULD:

Have cylinders hydrostatically tested at least once every 5 years

Have cylinders visually inspected annually

Use only clean, filtered air from an appropriate scuba fill station

Be aware that depth gauges are sometimes inaccurate, and have them tested periodically

Use proper and well-maintained equipment for all planned dives

Have my regulator and other safety devices checked and tested periodically

Know my boat and appropriate boating regulations

Use a diver's flag and surface support

Have a submersible pressure gauge to monitor tank air pressure

Dive with an alternative air source

Wear a buoyancy control device

Use an inflator on my BC

Have a dive-timing device

Ensure that the weight belt is not impeded by other equipment

AS A SAFE DIVER, I SHOULD:

Always test all my scuba equipment for proper fit/function

Plan my dive according to seas, actual weather, weather forecast, and my current physical condition

Have a dive plan that includes where and how to obtain emergency assistance

Be familiar with the dive site and determine whether it is a beginner or advanced site

Cancel dives when environmental conditions are questionable

Avoid touching anything underwater that may be alive

Remove any game killed in the water as soon as possible

Obey all local fish/game rules

RESTRICTIONS: AS A SAFE DIVER, I SHOULD:

Dive often

Never let an uncertified diver use my equipment

Never scuba dive with individuals who are not certified

Be aware of the effects of nitrogen narcosis on my ability to make judgment decisions

Obtain an orientation before diving in an unfamiliar area

Never dive below 100 feet

DIVE REVIEW: AS A SAFE DIVER, I SHOULD:

Strive to improve my diving knowledge by attending diving educational seminars and conventions

Have one or more reviews with a scuba instructor if it has been over 12 months since my last scuba dive, and have my logbook signed to show that I have dived within 12 months and I am competent in my scuba skills

GOOD CITIZEN: AS A SAFE DIVER, I SHOULD:

Be familiar with and obey all local diving laws

Be a good sportsman and obey all fish and game laws

I have read and understand the Sport Diver Standards for Safe Diving

---

Signature/Date

Appendix B

COURSE CRITIQUE

Your instructor would like to know how you feel about the course. Please complete this form and return it to your instructor. Your input will help your instructor improve the course for future students.

Name (Optional) _____

Course _____

Instructor _____

Class Number _____

Dates from _____ to _____

Check the appropriate box.	Poor	Fair	Average	Good	Excellent
1. Rate the overall course	☐	☐	☐	☐	☐
2. Rate the classroom sessions	☐	☐	☐	☐	☐
3. Rate the confined water/ pool sessions	☐	☐	☐	☐	☐
4. Rate the openwater dives	☐	☐	☐	☐	☐
5. Rate your instructor on the following:					
a. Knowledge	☐	☐	☐	☐	☐
b. Skill	☐	☐	☐	☐	☐
c. Organization	☐	☐	☐	☐	☐
d. Safety	☐	☐	☐	☐	☐
e. Starting on time	☐	☐	☐	☐	☐
f. Ending on time	☐	☐	☐	☐	☐
g. Staying on the subject	☐	☐	☐	☐	☐
h. Ability to relieve student apprehension and fear	☐	☐	☐	☐	☐

Write your response in the appropriate space.

6. Describe your impression of the course.

_____

_____

_____

7. Did the course meet your expectations? If not, explain why.

_____

_____

_____

8. What part of the course did you enjoy the most?

_____

_____

_____

9. What part of the course did you least enjoy?

_____

_____

_____

10. More time should be spent on

_____

_____

_____

11. Too much time was spent on

_____

_____

_____

12. The course could be improved by

_____

_____

_____

13. Where did you hear about this course?

_____

_____

14. Additional comments

_____

_____

_____

_____

_____

Appendix C

dive profile

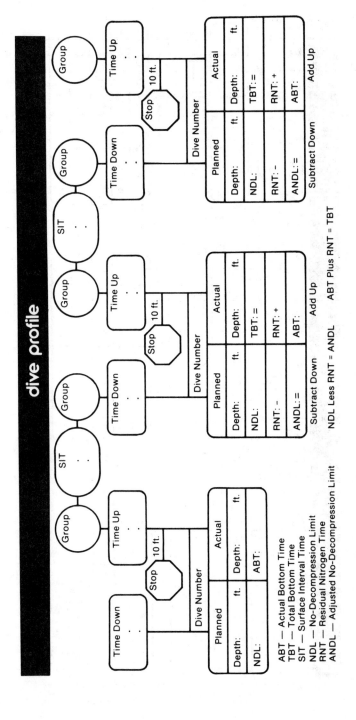

ABT — Actual Bottom Time
TBT — Total Bottom Time
SIT — Surface Interval Time
NDL — No-Decompression Limit
RNT — Residual Nitrogen Time
ANDL — Adjusted No-Decompression Limit

dive profile

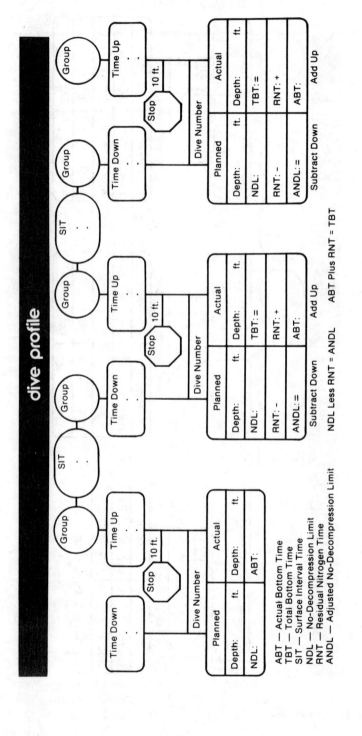

ABT — Actual Bottom Time
TBT — Total Bottom Time
SIT — Surface Interval Time
NDL — No-Decompression Limit
RNT — Residual Nitrogen Time
ANDL — Adjusted No-Decompression Limit

Subtract Down   Add Up   ABT Plus RNT = TBT

NDL Less RNT = ANDL

Appendix D

Chapter 1

1. a. mask
   b. fins
   c. snorkel
2. as small as possible
3. scuba
4. a. hypoallergenic
   b. ozone
5. a. heat
   b. facial oils
6. fit, comfort
7. tempered safety glass
8. a. noncorrosive
   b. removable
9. strong, positive locking
10. removing water
11. skirt
12. exhale gently
13. condense
14. before
15. abort
16. a. full-foot
    b. open-heel
17. b.
18. a. size
    b. leg
    c. conditions
19. a.
20. a. rub
    b. chafe
    c. off
    d. cramps
21. protect
22. a. flutter
    b. scissors
    c. frog
    d. dolphin
23. conserve air, surveying, area

24. rigid, flexible
25. a. breathing resistence
    b. comfort
26. mouthpiece
27. silicone
28. blasting or popping, expansion or displacement method
29. easy, safe, disorienting
30. giant stride
31. back-roll
32. donning, shuffling
33. kelp
34. look up, turn

Chapter 2

1. a. lycra dive skins
   b. wet suits
   c. dry suits
2. thermal, coral, barnacles
3. 25
4. buoyancy
5. correct fit
6. 3, 8, 6, 5, 1, 9, 4, 7, 2
7. 6
8. release, right
9. under
10. a. neck, wrists
    b. zipper
    c. boots
11. a. extremely cold
    b. bottom times, moderately
12. sink slightly, rise slightly
13. nylon web
14. release
15. boat, pool
16. see it drop
17. skin divers (diving)
18. waist, arms

19. double bag
20. single bag
21. buoyancy compensation device
22. inflating, submerging

Chapter 3

1. young, lightweight
2. steel, aluminum
3. galvanized
4. illegal
5. 3000
6. K (non-reserve)
7. J
8. "O"-ring
9. quick-release
10. tank band
11. moisture
12. low
13. annually
14. white
15. does not
16. nothing
17. 5
18. 2
19. single, two-stage
20. breathing ease, durability, dependability
21. octopus
22. buddy breathing
23. primary second stage
24. first, second, air supply
25. regularly
26. purge button
27. exhale
28. blasting, purge button
29. one
30. eye
31. exhale continuously
32. stop your ascent
33. find, operate
34. stay together, signals, emergency
35. within arm's reach

Chapter 4

1. SPG
2. head, numbers, glass
3. regularly monitoring, consumption, remaining
4. water-resistant, waterproof
5. relatively shallow
6. a. capillary
   b. bourdon tube
   c. diaphragm
   d. electronic
7. capillary
8. maximum depth needle
9. depth, time
10. operation manual
11. dive computer
12. dive conservatively
13. no-decompression dives
14. ascent rate
15. 10, 30, 3, 5
16. deepest
17. your computer off
18. failure
19. flying
20. convenience, safety
21. compass
22. wrist
23. a. 360 (O)
    b. 90
    c. 180
    d. 270
24. level
25. 180
26. kelp, grass
27. ripple marks

Chapter 5

1. visible
2. alpha
3. whistle
4. chemical light sticks

5. a. hammer
   b. saw
   c. screwdriver
   d. lever
   e. pry bar
   f. ruler
   g. probe
   h. cutting tool
6. fishing line
7. sealed
8. sealed beam
9. waterproof, pressure proof
10. planning future dives
11. repetitive dive
12. logbook
13. tools, spare parts
14. tank, weight belt

Chapter 6

1. positive buoyancy
2. negatively buoyant
3. neutrally buoyant
4. salt water
5. bigger, closer
6. reds, oranges
7. 4
8. signals
9. 25
10. terminate

Chapter 7

1. 78
2. inert
3. carbon dioxide
4. stop, rest, breathe deeply
5. 3, 4
6. a. wide eyed
   b. rapid
   c. action
7. stop, think, breathe slowly, deeply

8. mouth, mouth
9. cardiac massage
10. CPR
11. open the, airway
12. pulse
13. pocket mask
14. clean, dry, filtered
15. diving air

Chapter 8

1. 14.7
2. 33
3. 34
4. absolute
5. 3
6. 1/2
7. 2
8. a. ears
   b. sinuses
   c. lungs, airways
   d. stomach
   e. intestines
9. middle ear
10. sinus squeeze
11. air embolism
12. a. flat
    b. CPR
    c. 100% oxygen
    d. 100% oxygen
    e. shock
    f. recompression chamber
13. 919-684-8111
14. HOLD YOUR BREATH
15. 33, 100
16. your buddy
17. head
18. 60
19. 3
20. OK
21. out of air
22. buddy breathing
23. weight belt

Chapter 9

1. 100
2. 30
3. narcosis, 60
4. 2
5. oxygen
6. oxygen toxicity
7. nitrogen
8. slowly
9. 10
10. first hour
11. 36
12. a. joint
    b. rash
    c. numbness, tingling
    d. personality
    e. fatigue
    f. vision
    g. weakness
13. 60
14. Any of the following: age, fatigue, alcohol use, drug use, old injuries, dehydration, hot showers after diving, tight-fitting dive suits, obesity
15. pregnancy
16. 60
17. 15
18. descent, ascent directly
19. 2300
20. 12, 24

Chapter 10

1. 24, saturated
2. nitrogen
3. 10, 20
4. residual
5. depth
6. repetitive dive
7. profile
8. surface interval time, SIT
9. USN: 60
   Jeppesen: 50
   DCIEM: 50
   NAUI('90): 55
   PADI-RDP('89): 55
10. USN: H
    Jeppesen: H
    DCIEM: F
    NAUI('90): H
    PADI-RDP('89): U
11. USN: 37
    Jeppesen: 290
    DCIEM: 180 (rf =1. 3)
    NAUI('90): 102
    PADI-RDP('89): 51
12. USN: D
    Jeppesen: D
    DCIEM: 1. 3 (B equivalent)
    NAUI('90): D
    PADI-RDP('89): A
13. USN: 29
    Jeppesen: 29
    DCIEM: N/A (25 computed by interpolation)
    NAUI('90): 29
    PADI-RDP('89): 7
14. USN: J
    Jeppesen: J
    DCIEM: G
    NAUI('90): J
    PADI-RDP('90): R
15. USN: 2300
    Jeppesen: 2300
    DCIEM: 999 (Up to10,000 with Table D)
    NAUI('90): 1000
    PADI-RDP('89): 1000
16. USN: 60
    Jeppesen: 60
    DCIEM: 60
    NAUI('90): 60
    PADI-RDP('89): 60
17. Decompression sickness (DCS)
18. USN: H, D, 37, I
    Jeppesen: H, D, 37, I
    DCIEM: F*, 1. 4**, 24, G (* = decompression dive, ** = C equivalent)
    NAUI('90): H, D, 37, I
    PADI-RDP('89): T, B,16, R

Chapter 11

1. 70. 8
2. continental shelf
3. ecology
4. water temperature
5. 64
6. thermoclines
7. overturn
8. upwelling
9. airmass
10. frontal, front
11. National Weather
12. NOAA
    a. 162. 550
    b. 162. 400
    c. 162. 475
13. cloud, wind, temperature
14. saturated
15. falling

Chapter 12

1. bulges, moon, sun
2. high tide
3. stand
4. range
5. tidal flat
6. tidal current
7. flood
8. ebb
9. slack
10. circular
11. clockwise, counterclockwise
12. wind, geologic
13. velocity
14. fetch
15. sea
16. height
17. crest, crest
18. reef, sandbar
19. backrush
20. surge
21. longshore
22. rip
23. into
24. whistle

Chapter 13

1. hard, soft
2. sexually, asexually
3. relatively shallow, warm
4. symbiotic
5. animal
6. 20, 40
7. 75, 30, 30
8. eastern
9. rocks, kelp
10. algae
11. parrotfish
12. starfish, shellfish
13. bait, dead fish
14. barracuda
15. moray eel
16. shuffle
17. avoid
18. a. size
    b. speed
    c. camouflage
    d. barbs
    e. stingers
    f. teeth

Chapter 14

1. sandpits, quarries, caves, sinkholes, springs
2. overhead
3. 18
4. natural
5. rivers
6. sinkholes, springs
7. freshwater
8. frogs, toads, newts, salamanders
9. turtles, snakes, alligators

10. man
11. manatee

Chapter 15

1. symbiosis
2. sewage, garbage
3. Red Tide
4. silt
5. oil
6. over-harvesting
7. food
8. eutrophication
9. acid rain
10. pollution

Chapter 16

1. overfishing
2. sport
3. Hawaiian sling
4. a. fish
   b. area
5. load, unload
6. 2
7. die, eaten
8. conch
9. spiny
10. Maine
11. crabs
12. turtle, salmon, shrimp, oyster
13. seaweed

Chapter 17

1. planning
2. conditioning
3. nutrition
4. fats, oils
5. whole grains, rice, fruit, vegetables
6. hydration
7. urine

8. a. coffee
   b. cola
   c. tea
   d. alcohol
9. conservatively
10. plan
11. site
12. a. depths
    b. expected visibility
    c. hazards
    d. local surfs
    e. tides
    f. currents
    g. bottom type and composition
    h. underwater life
13. emergency, emergency
14. equipment checklist
15. dive
16. week
17. dive plan
18. dive your plan
19. cancel
20. 60, 40
21. 100

Chapter 18

1. southeast
2. mines, quarries
3. sinkhole
4. cavern
5. 130
6. restrictions
7. 40
8. 70
9. decompression
10. cave
11. cave diving
12. artifacts
13. prospecting
14. bottom, deeper
15. buoyancy control
16. down line
17. tether

18. law enforcement
19. NASAR

Chapter 19

1. instructor
2. journalism
3. education, adventure, travel
4. photography
5. short, decompression
6. imagination
7. training
8. paid, dangerous
9. welding, hard, mixed gas
10. AAUS
11. oceanography, limnology